Reversing Eosinophilic Esophagitis

The Raw Vegan Detoxification & Regeneration Workbook for Curing Patients.

Global Healing

Copyright © 2023

All rights reserved. Without limiting rights under the copyright reserved above, no part of this publication may be reproduced, stored, introduced into a retrieval system, distributed or transmitted in any form or by any means, including without limitation photocopying, recording, or other electronic or mechanical methods, without the prior written permission of the publisher, except in the case of brief quotations embodied in critical reviews and certain other non-commercial uses permitted by copyright law.

This book, with the opinions, suggestions and references made within it, is based on the author's personal experience and is for personal study and research purposes only. This program is about health and vitality, not disease. The author makes no medical claims. If you choose to use the material in this book on yourself, the author and publisher take no responsibility for your actions and decisions or the consequences thereof..

The scanning, uploading, and/or distribution of this document via the internet or via any other means without the permission of the publisher is illegal and is punishable by law. Please purchase only authorized editions and do not participate in or encourage electronic piracy of copyrightable materials

Introduction & Summary

"Let food be thy medicine and medicine be thy food."
- Hippocrates

In order to deliver you the maximum benefit in the shortest time possible, we have refrained from writing up an information-overloaded book. Instead, within this short section, we will summarise the key points that we have discovered through our work with Eosinophilic Esophagitis patients.

It is common knowledge that the food we consume on a daily basis directly relates to both our physical and mental health. Acid forming foods (mainly animal and starch based cooked foods) create the ideal environment within our bodies for an dis-ease/imbalance to exist. An alkaline environment (achieved mainly through raw plant-based foods - predominantly fruits) within the body repels disease, suffering and pain, while healing and regenerating.

Having healed numerous patients – we have come to a series of conclusions and treatment protocols;

1. Whatever the labelled "condition" or "disease" is – the hindrance of an internal acidic environment can be corrected. If your car had an oil leak, you wouldn't just seal the leak, you would find the root of it and fix this. Similarly we want to correct the root causes for real results.

2. In simple terms, "dis-ease" within the body stems from internal congestion. It can also be referred to as constipation, a stagnant lymphatic system, an acidic state, excessive internal mucus, lazy kidneys, or slow bowel movements.

3. The key to healing is to cleanse the two fluids found within the human body (blood and lymph). The lymphatic system's fluid serves as the blood's washing system and carries its waste out of the body through the three kidneys (your skin being the 3rd kidney – through sweat/deep heat/sauna). Having regular bowel movements also supports the detoxification process.

4. Sleep, sleep and more sleep. Good quality and regular sleep is extremely important – this is your body's opportunity to repair and recover. During your healing period, aim for at least 8 hours of sleep, and stop all consumption by the evening so your body can start it's recovery phase of the day (as nature intended).

5. Dry fasting supports the body in eliminating toxins and cells that are not performing at their best. Intermittent fasting has helped many patients achieve positive results. **Avoid if pregnant**: Dry fast until as late as possible into the day before eating a fruit that has a laxative effect (e.g. prunes, plums, grapes, figs, oranges). This process will help flush out the fast's resulting toxins. Note: after a long dry fast, a laxative fruit is necessary because fasts can cause constipation.

6. The longer you can dry fast, the better the results will be. However, you must work up to this. Don't just jump in with a long dry fast, especially if you have weak kidneys. Start by having a delayed fruit breakfast, working towards skipping breakfast altogether, to having only 1 fruit meal in the day. **Always work at your own pace**.

7. This protocol becomes easier with time. Your first week of dry fasting with fruits can be challenging but your body adapts and eventually it is second nature. The vitality that you will feel within yourself will motivate you to carry on. The key is to complete 7 consecutive days of fruit fasting (it becomes significantly easier from this point on) and then to 14 days, 30 days, and so on.

8. Fruit (melons, berries, grapes) with the rich fructose content will be your main food during your detoxification period. **For the deepest detox experience**, slow juice your fruits and stick with a single fruit throughout (grape juice alone has given us the best results).

9. Juicing allows for accelerated results (your body can focus all of its energy on healing as opposed to digestion). Certain herbs (e.g. Parsley, Cilantro) will enhance detoxification. Vegetables tend to slow down the detoxification process, while starches, nuts/seeds, legumes, and cooked foods will halt the detoxification process.

Note: Proteins, dairy, and grain based foods will reverse your detoxification progress so these foods need to be eliminated from your diet during your healing phase.

10. Dried fruits (dates, figs, apricots, bananas, avocados) can be used to assist if you are feeling empty or struggling in the initial stages. However, do get back onto water dense fresh fruit (watermelons/melons, berries, oranges, and grapes being the preferred kind) as soon as possible (ideally juiced). A list of detox-proven fruits can be found in the following point.

11. Examples of fruits proven to offer reliable detoxification: Apples, Apricots, Blueberries, Blackberries, Cherries, Clementines, Figs, Tangerines, Lemons, Limes, Grapefruit, Mango, Grapes, Strawberries, Raspberries, Oranges, Pomegranates, Pineapples, Plums, Pears, Prunes, Watermelon

12. Keep up your water intake throughout the day. Water from a spring is ideal (mineral rich).

13. If you are on medications, work with your Medical Doctor (MD) and have regular blood work done so your personal progress can be monitored. **Positive results will occur within a short timeframe** so do pay close attention to your state and remember to reduce medication if no longer required.

Our goal throughout this workbook is to help you with recording your progress and applying the information stated in the above points.

Start with what you are most comfortable with and make it enjoyable, choose your favourite sweet fruits. If a client deviates from the routine, we advise to get back on track as soon as possible. Just keep moving forward and be persistent. Never give up!

We would like to wish you all the best and if you have any questions, thoughts, or comments, feel free to email us at:

HealingCentral8@gmail.com

Good Luck with your journey.

[EXAMPLE 1]
Today's Date: 6th May 2018

Morning
I just ate 3 mangoes – very sweet and tasty. I felt a heavy feeling under my chest area so I stopped eating. Unsure what that was – maybe digestive or the transverse colon?

Afternoon
I was feeling hungry so I am eating some dried figs, pineapple and apricots with around 750ml of spring water.

Evening
Sipping on a green tea (herbal). Feeling pretty strong and alert at the moment.

Night
Enjoying a bowl of red seeded grapes. Currently I feel satisfied.

Today's Notes (Highlights, Thoughts, Feelings):

Unlike yesterday, today was a good day. I am noticing an increase in regular bowel movements which makes me feel cleansed and light afterwards. I feel as though my kidneys are also starting to filter better (white sediment visible in morning wee).

It definitely helps to document my thoughts in this workbook. A great way to reflect, improve and stay on track.

Feeling very good – vibrant and strong – I have noticed a major improvement in my physical fitness and performance. Mentally I feel healthier and happier.

[EXAMPLE 2]
Today's Date: 7th May 2018

Morning
Dry fasting (water and food free since 8pm last night) - will go up until 12:30pm today, and start with 500ml of spring water before eating half a watermelon.

Afternoon
Kept busy and was in and out quite a bit - so nothing consumed.

Evening
At around 5pm, I had a peppermint tea with a selection of mixed dried fruit (small bowl of apricot, dates, mango, pineapple, and prunes).

Night
Sipped on spring water through the evening as required.
Finished off the other half of the watermelon from the morning.

Today's Notes (Highlights, Thoughts, Feelings):

As with most days, today started well with me dry fasting (continuing my fast from my sleep/skipping breakfast) up until around 12:30pm and then eating half a watermelon. The laxative effect of the watermelon helped me poop and release any loosened toxins from the fasting period.
I tend to struggle on some days from 3pm onwards. Up until that point I am okay but if the cravings strike then it can be challenging. I remind myself that those burgers and chips do not have any live healing energy.
I feel good in general. I feel fantastic doing a fruit/juice fast but slightly empty by the end of the day.
Cooked food makes me feel severe fatigue and mental fog.
Will continue with my fruit fasting and start to introduce fruit juices due to their deeper detox benefits. I would love to be on juices only as I have seen others within the community achieve amazing results.

[EXAMPLE 3]
Today's Date: 8th May 2018

Morning
Today I woke and my children were enjoying some watermelon for breakfast - and the smell was luring so I joined them. Large bowl of watermelon eaten at around 8am. Started with a glass of water.

Afternoon
Snacked on left over watermelon throughout the morning and afternoon. Had 5 dates an hour or so after.

Evening
Had around 3 mangoes at around 6pm. Felt content - but then I was invited round to a family gathering where a selection of pizzas, burgers and chips were being served. I gave into the peer pressure and felt like I let myself down!

Night
Having over-eaten earlier on in the evening, I was still feeling bloated with a headache (possibly digestion related) and I also felt quite mucus filled (wheez in chest and coughing up phlegm). Very sleepy and low energy. The perils of cooked foods!!

Today's Notes (Highlights, Thoughts, Feelings):

I let myself down today. It all started well until I ate a fully blown meal (and over-ate). I didn't remain focussed and I spun off track. As a result my energy levels were much lower and I felt a bout of extreme fatigue 30 minutes after the meal (most likely the body struggling to with digesting all that cooked food).
I need to stick to the plan because the difference between fruit fasting, and eating cooked foods is huge - 1 makes you feel empowered whilst the other makes you feel drained. I also felt the mucus overload after the meal - it kicked in pretty quickly.
Today I felt disappointed after giving in to the meal but tomorrow is a new day and I will keep on going! It is important to remind myself that I won't get better if I cannot stick to the routine.

Today's Date:

Morning
(work towards continuing your night time dry fast up until at least 12pm)

Afternoon
(get hydrating with fresh fruit or even better slow juiced fruits/berries/melons)

Evening
(aim to wind down to a dry fast by around 6pm to 7pm)

Night
(work your way up to dry fasting from the evening until 12pm the following day)

Today's Notes (Highlights, Thoughts, Feelings, What Could You Improve On?)

"Get yourself an accountability partner to complete a 3 month detox with. Start with 7 days and work your way up. It will be fun and motivating completing it with somebody (or a group) ...or of course you can go it alone"

Today's Date:

Morning
(work towards continuing your night time dry fast up until at least 12pm)

Afternoon
(get hydrating with fresh fruit or even better slow juiced fruits/berries/melons)

Evening
(aim to wind down to a dry fast by around 6pm to 7pm)

Night
(work your way up to dry fasting from the evening until 12pm the following day)

Today's Notes (Highlights, Thoughts, Feelings, What Could You Improve On?)

"Remember to keep yourself hydrated with water too (spring water preferred)."

Today's Date:

Morning
(work towards continuing your night time dry fast up until at least 12pm)

Afternoon
(get hydrating with fresh fruit or even better slow juiced fruits/berries/melons)

Evening
(aim to wind down to a dry fast by around 6pm to 7pm)

Night
(work your way up to dry fasting from the evening until 12pm the following day)

Today's Notes (Highlights, Thoughts, Feelings, What Could You Improve On?)

"Eat melons/watermelons separately, and before any other fruit as it digests faster and we want to limit fermentation (acidity) which can occur if other fruits are mixed in."

Today's Date:

Morning
(work towards continuing your night time dry fast up until at least 12pm)

Afternoon
(get hydrating with fresh fruit or even better slow juiced fruits/berries/melons)

Evening
(aim to wind down to a dry fast by around 6pm to 7pm)

Night
(work your way up to dry fasting from the evening until 12pm the following day)

Today's Notes (Highlights, Thoughts, Feelings, What Could You Improve On?)

"Stay focussed on the end goal of removing mucus & toxins from your body and feeling wonderful again!"

Today's Date:

Morning
(work towards continuing your night time dry fast up until at least 12pm)

Afternoon
(get hydrating with fresh fruit or even better slow juiced fruits/berries/melons)

Evening
(aim to wind down to a dry fast by around 6pm to 7pm)

Night
(work your way up to dry fasting from the evening until 12pm the following day)

Today's Notes (Highlights, Thoughts, Feelings, What Could You Improve On?)

"Meditate and perform deep breathing exercises in order to help yourself remain present minded and stay on track."

Today's Date:

Morning
(work towards continuing your night time dry fast up until at least 12pm)

Afternoon
(get hydrating with fresh fruit or even better slow juiced fruits/berries/melons)

Evening
(aim to wind down to a dry fast by around 6pm to 7pm)

Night
(work your way up to dry fasting from the evening until 12pm the following day)

Today's Notes (Highlights, Thoughts, Feelings, What Could You Improve On?)

"Join a few like-minded communities – there are many juicing and raw vegan based groups, both online and offline. Being part of a community can help motivate you to reach your goals."

Today's Date:

Morning
(work towards continuing your night time dry fast up until at least 12pm)

Afternoon
(get hydrating with fresh fruit or even better slow juiced fruits/berries/melons)

Evening
(aim to wind down to a dry fast by around 6pm to 7pm)

Night
(work your way up to dry fasting from the evening until 12pm the following day)

Today's Notes (Highlights, Thoughts, Feelings, What Could You Improve On?)

"If you are struggling with hunger pangs in the early stages, try some dates or dried apricots, prunes, or raisins, with a cup of herbal tea.

Today's Date:

Morning
(work towards continuing your night time dry fast up until at least 12pm)

Afternoon
(get hydrating with fresh fruit or even better slow juiced fruits/berries/melons)

Evening
(aim to wind down to a dry fast by around 6pm to 7pm)

Night
(work your way up to dry fasting from the evening until 12pm the following day)

Today's Notes (Highlights, Thoughts, Feelings, What Could You Improve On?)

"Get into a routine of regularly buying fresh fruit (or grow your own if weather permits) to keep your supplies up."

Today's Date:

Morning
(work towards continuing your night time dry fast up until at least 12pm)

Afternoon
(get hydrating with fresh fruit or even better slow juiced fruits/berries/melons)

Evening
(aim to wind down to a dry fast by around 6pm to 7pm)

Night
(work your way up to dry fasting from the evening until 12pm the following day)

Today's Notes (Highlights, Thoughts, Feelings, What Could You Improve On?)

"Regularly remind yourself about the great rewards and benefits that you will experience from keeping up this detox."

Today's Date:

────────────────── **Morning** ──────────────────
(work towards continuing your night time dry fast up until at least 12pm)

────────────────── **Afternoon** ──────────────────
(get hydrating with fresh fruit or even better slow juiced fruits/berries/melons)

────────────────── **Evening** ──────────────────
(aim to wind down to a dry fast by around 6pm to 7pm)

────────────────── **Night** ──────────────────
(work your way up to dry fasting from the evening until 12pm the following day)

Today's Notes (Highlights, Thoughts, Feelings, What Could You Improve On?)

"Keep your teeth brushed and flossed regularly – at least twice a day to keep them healthy for your fruit sessions. You will notice an improvement in your dental health with this raw/fruit diet."

Today's Date:

―――――――――――― **Morning** ――――――――――――
(work towards continuing your night time dry fast up until at least 12pm)

―――――――――――― **Afternoon** ――――――――――――
(get hydrating with fresh fruit or even better slow juiced fruits/berries/melons)

―――――――――――― **Evening** ――――――――――――
(aim to wind down to a dry fast by around 6pm to 7pm)

―――――――――――― **Night** ――――――――――――
(work your way up to dry fasting from the evening until 12pm the following day)

Today's Notes (Highlights, Thoughts, Feelings, What Could You Improve On?)

"Be motivated by the vision of becoming an example for others to learn from and follow."

Today's Date:

Morning
(work towards continuing your night time dry fast up until at least 12pm)

Afternoon
(get hydrating with fresh fruit or even better slow juiced fruits/berries/melons)

Evening
(aim to wind down to a dry fast by around 6pm to 7pm)

Night
(work your way up to dry fasting from the evening until 12pm the following day)

Today's Notes (Highlights, Thoughts, Feelings, What Could You Improve On?)

"Embrace your achievements and wonderful results – feel and appreciate the difference within you as a result of this new routine."

Today's Date:

Morning
(work towards continuing your night time dry fast up until at least 12pm)

Afternoon
(get hydrating with fresh fruit or even better slow juiced fruits/berries/melons)

Evening
(aim to wind down to a dry fast by around 6pm to 7pm)

Night
(work your way up to dry fasting from the evening until 12pm the following day)

Today's Notes (Highlights, Thoughts, Feelings, What Could You Improve On?)

"Buy fruit in bulk where possible so you have ample supplies for a week or two in advance. If in a hot climate, you could even freeze your fruit or make ice lollies out of it (crush & freeze)."

Today's Date:

―――――――――――― **Morning** ――――――――――――
(work towards continuing your night time dry fast up until at least 12pm)

―――――――――――― **Afternoon** ――――――――――――
(get hydrating with fresh fruit or even better slow juiced fruits/berries/melons)

―――――――――――― **Evening** ――――――――――――
(aim to wind down to a dry fast by around 6pm to 7pm)

―――――――――――― **Night** ――――――――――――
(work your way up to dry fasting from the evening until 12pm the following day)

Today's Notes (Highlights, Thoughts, Feelings, What Could You Improve On?)

"Stay as busy as you can during the daytime. Creating a busy routine makes it easier to manage your diet."

Today's Date:

Morning
(work towards continuing your night time dry fast up until at least 12pm)

Afternoon
(get hydrating with fresh fruit or even better slow juiced fruits/berries/melons)

Evening
(aim to wind down to a dry fast by around 6pm to 7pm)

Night
(work your way up to dry fasting from the evening until 12pm the following day)

Today's Notes (Highlights, Thoughts, Feelings, What Could You Improve On?)

"Complete your fruit and fasting routine with a group of friends/family/colleagues so you can all support one another."

Today's Date:

Morning
(work towards continuing your night time dry fast up until at least 12pm)

Afternoon
(get hydrating with fresh fruit or even better slow juiced fruits/berries/melons)

Evening
(aim to wind down to a dry fast by around 6pm to 7pm)

Night
(work your way up to dry fasting from the evening until 12pm the following day)

Today's Notes (Highlights, Thoughts, Feelings, What Could You Improve On?)

"Monitor your urine regularly. Urinate in a jar and leave overnight. If you see a thick cloud of white sediment (success!), your kidneys are filtering acids out."

Today's Date:

———————————— **Morning** ————————————
(work towards continuing your night time dry fast up until at least 12pm)

———————————— **Afternoon** ————————————
(get hydrating with fresh fruit or even better slow juiced fruits/berries/melons)

———————————— **Evening** ————————————
(aim to wind down to a dry fast by around 6pm to 7pm)

———————————— **Night** ————————————
(work your way up to dry fasting from the evening until 12pm the following day)

Today's Notes (Highlights, Thoughts, Feelings, What Could You Improve On?)

"Have genuine love and care for yourself. If craving junk food, affirm positive inner talk ("if I eat this, I won't feel good so leave it out")".

Today's Date:

Morning
(work towards continuing your night time dry fast up until at least 12pm)

Afternoon
(get hydrating with fresh fruit or even better slow juiced fruits/berries/melons)

Evening
(aim to wind down to a dry fast by around 6pm to 7pm)

Night
(work your way up to dry fasting from the evening until 12pm the following day)

Today's Notes (Highlights, Thoughts, Feelings, What Could You Improve On?)

"Filter out unwanted acids with this alkaline water-dense fruits protocol."

Today's Date:

―――――――――――――― **Morning** ――――――――――――――
(work towards continuing your night time dry fast up until at least 12pm)

―――――――――――――― **Afternoon** ――――――――――――――
(get hydrating with fresh fruit or even better slow juiced fruits/berries/melons)

―――――――――――――― **Evening** ――――――――――――――
(aim to wind down to a dry fast by around 6pm to 7pm)

―――――――――――――― **Night** ――――――――――――――
(work your way up to dry fasting from the evening until 12pm the following day)

Today's Notes (Highlights, Thoughts, Feelings, What Could You Improve On?)

"Look out for white cloud/sediment (acids) in your urine to confirm kidney filtration."

Today's Date:

———————————— Morning ————————————
(work towards continuing your night time dry fast up until at least 12pm)

———————————— Afternoon ————————————
(get hydrating with fresh fruit or even better slow juiced fruits/berries/melons)

———————————— Evening ————————————
(aim to wind down to a dry fast by around 6pm to 7pm)

———————————— Night ————————————
(work your way up to dry fasting from the evening until 12pm the following day)

Today's Notes (Highlights, Thoughts, Feelings, What Could You Improve On?)

"Infections emerge in an acidic environment"

Today's Date:

Morning
(work towards continuing your night time dry fast up until at least 12pm)

Afternoon
(get hydrating with fresh fruit or even better slow juiced fruits/berries/melons)

Evening
(aim to wind down to a dry fast by around 6pm to 7pm)

Night
(work your way up to dry fasting from the evening until 12pm the following day)

Today's Notes (Highlights, Thoughts, Feelings, What Could You Improve On?)

"Any deficiencies that you may have will disappear once you have cleansed your clogged up gut/colon, kidneys and various other eliminative organs."

Today's Date:

Morning
(work towards continuing your night time dry fast up until at least 12pm)

Afternoon
(get hydrating with fresh fruit or even better slow juiced fruits/berries/melons)

Evening
(aim to wind down to a dry fast by around 6pm to 7pm)

Night
(work your way up to dry fasting from the evening until 12pm the following day)

Today's Notes (Highlights, Thoughts, Feelings, What Could You Improve On?)

"Dependant on how deeply you detox yourself, you could even eliminate any genetic weaknesses that you may have inherited."

Today's Date:

─────────────── **Morning** ───────────────

(work towards continuing your night time dry fast up until at least 12pm)

─────────────── **Afternoon** ───────────────

(get hydrating with fresh fruit or even better slow juiced fruits/berries/melons)

─────────────── **Evening** ───────────────

(aim to wind down to a dry fast by around 6pm to 7pm)

─────────────── **Night** ───────────────

(work your way up to dry fasting from the evening until 12pm the following day)

Today's Notes (Highlights, Thoughts, Feelings, What Could You Improve On?)

"Keep focused on your detox. Even past injuries / trauma are all repairable for good."

Today's Date:

Morning
(work towards continuing your night time dry fast up until at least 12pm)

Afternoon
(get hydrating with fresh fruit or even better slow juiced fruits/berries/melons)

Evening
(aim to wind down to a dry fast by around 6pm to 7pm)

Night
(work your way up to dry fasting from the evening until 12pm the following day)

Today's Notes (Highlights, Thoughts, Feelings, What Could You Improve On?)

"If you suffer from ongoing sadness / depression, a deep detox will support your mental health. You will soon notice a positive change in your mood."

Today's Date:

──────────────── **Morning** ────────────────
(work towards continuing your night time dry fast up until at least 12pm)

──────────────── **Afternoon** ────────────────
(get hydrating with fresh fruit or even better slow juiced fruits/berries/melons)

──────────────── **Evening** ────────────────
(aim to wind down to a dry fast by around 6pm to 7pm)

──────────────── **Night** ────────────────
(work your way up to dry fasting from the evening until 12pm the following day)

Today's Notes (Highlights, Thoughts, Feelings, What Could You Improve On?)

"Have your fruits/juices throughout the day. As the evening approaches, start to dry fast – your body wants to rest and heal from this point on."

Today's Date:

Morning
(work towards continuing your night time dry fast up until at least 12pm)

Afternoon
(get hydrating with fresh fruit or even better slow juiced fruits/berries/melons)

Evening
(aim to wind down to a dry fast by around 6pm to 7pm)

Night
(work your way up to dry fasting from the evening until 12pm the following day)

Today's Notes (Highlights, Thoughts, Feelings, What Could You Improve On?)

"The kidneys dislike proteins but really appreciate juicy fruits like melons, berries, citrus fruits, pineapples, mangoes, apples, grapes."

Today's Date:

———————————— **Morning** ————————————
(work towards continuing your night time dry fast up until at least 12pm)

———————————— **Afternoon** ————————————
(get hydrating with fresh fruit or even better slow juiced fruits/berries/melons)

———————————— **Evening** ————————————
(aim to wind down to a dry fast by around 6pm to 7pm)

———————————— **Night** ————————————
(work your way up to dry fasting from the evening until 12pm the following day)

Today's Notes (Highlights, Thoughts, Feelings, What Could You Improve On?)

"Healing is very easy. There's no need to complicate it. Keep it simple and you will see results."

Today's Date:

Morning
(work towards continuing your night time dry fast up until at least 12pm)

Afternoon
(get hydrating with fresh fruit or even better slow juiced fruits/berries/melons)

Evening
(aim to wind down to a dry fast by around 6pm to 7pm)

Night
(work your way up to dry fasting from the evening until 12pm the following day)

Today's Notes (Highlights, Thoughts, Feelings, What Could You Improve On?)

"Keep your body in an alkaline state as this is where regeneration takes place."

Today's Date:

Morning
(work towards continuing your night time dry fast up until at least 12pm)

Afternoon
(get hydrating with fresh fruit or even better slow juiced fruits/berries/melons)

Evening
(aim to wind down to a dry fast by around 6pm to 7pm)

Night
(work your way up to dry fasting from the evening until 12pm the following day)

Today's Notes (Highlights, Thoughts, Feelings, What Could You Improve On?)

"A daily enema with boiled water (cooled down) will support your detox greatly."

Today's Date:

Morning
(work towards continuing your night time dry fast up until at least 12pm)

Afternoon
(get hydrating with fresh fruit or even better slow juiced fruits/berries/melons)

Evening
(aim to wind down to a dry fast by around 6pm to 7pm)

Night
(work your way up to dry fasting from the evening until 12pm the following day)

Today's Notes (Highlights, Thoughts, Feelings, What Could You Improve On?)

"Have your iris' read by an iridologist that works with Dr Bernard Jensen's system."

Today's Date:

―――――――――――――― **Morning** ――――――――――――――
(work towards continuing your night time dry fast up until at least 12pm)

―――――――――――――― **Afternoon** ――――――――――――――
(get hydrating with fresh fruit or even better slow juiced fruits/berries/melons)

―――――――――――――― **Evening** ――――――――――――――
(aim to wind down to a dry fast by around 6pm to 7pm)

―――――――――――――― **Night** ――――――――――――――
(work your way up to dry fasting from the evening until 12pm the following day)

Today's Notes (Highlights, Thoughts, Feelings, What Could You Improve On?)

"Take a herbal parasite formula for a month. It will eliminate food cravings. This is an important point."

Today's Date:

———————————— **Morning** ————————————
(work towards continuing your night time dry fast up until at least 12pm)

———————————— **Afternoon** ————————————
(get hydrating with fresh fruit or even better slow juiced fruits/berries/melons)

———————————— **Evening** ————————————
(aim to wind down to a dry fast by around 6pm to 7pm)

———————————— **Night** ————————————
(work your way up to dry fasting from the evening until 12pm the following day)

Today's Notes (Highlights, Thoughts, Feelings, What Could You Improve On?)

"Your skin is the largest eliminative organ. Skin brushing and sweating are crucial. Sauna heat is ideal, steam can also work."

Today's Date:

Morning
(work towards continuing your night time dry fast up until at least 12pm)

Afternoon
(get hydrating with fresh fruit or even better slow juiced fruits/berries/melons)

Evening
(aim to wind down to a dry fast by around 6pm to 7pm)

Night
(work your way up to dry fasting from the evening until 12pm the following day)

Today's Notes (Highlights, Thoughts, Feelings, What Could You Improve On?)

"If you are on medications, monitor the relevant statistics (e.g. blood pressure, blood sugar level, etc). Upon improving, lower medication"

Today's Date:

Morning
(work towards continuing your night time dry fast up until at least 12pm)

Afternoon
(get hydrating with fresh fruit or even better slow juiced fruits/berries/melons)

Evening
(aim to wind down to a dry fast by around 6pm to 7pm)

Night
(work your way up to dry fasting from the evening until 12pm the following day)

Today's Notes (Highlights, Thoughts, Feelings, What Could You Improve On?)

"Most people do not breathe effectively. Your body requires a healthy supply of oxygen to heal. Practice breathing techniques daily."

Today's Date:

Morning
(work towards continuing your night time dry fast up until at least 12pm)

Afternoon
(get hydrating with fresh fruit or even better slow juiced fruits/berries/melons)

Evening
(aim to wind down to a dry fast by around 6pm to 7pm)

Night
(work your way up to dry fasting from the evening until 12pm the following day)

Today's Notes (Highlights, Thoughts, Feelings, What Could You Improve On?)

"Disease is not the presence of something evil, but rather the lack of the presence of something essential."
— *Dr. Bernard Jensen.*

Today's Date:

Morning
(work towards continuing your night time dry fast up until at least 12pm)

Afternoon
(get hydrating with fresh fruit or even better slow juiced fruits/berries/melons)

Evening
(aim to wind down to a dry fast by around 6pm to 7pm)

Night
(work your way up to dry fasting from the evening until 12pm the following day)

Today's Notes (Highlights, Thoughts, Feelings, What Could You Improve On?)

"Fruits will empower you, providing live energy. Cooked foods in comparison will use vital energy that could otherwise be used for healing."

Today's Date:

Morning
(work towards continuing your night time dry fast up until at least 12pm)

Afternoon
(get hydrating with fresh fruit or even better slow juiced fruits/berries/melons)

Evening
(aim to wind down to a dry fast by around 6pm to 7pm)

Night
(work your way up to dry fasting from the evening until 12pm the following day)

Today's Notes (Highlights, Thoughts, Feelings, What Could You Improve On?)

"Fructose (the sugar found in fruits) is kind to the pancreas and its absorption into the body uses minimal energy."

Today's Date:

—————————————— **Morning** ——————————————
(work towards continuing your night time dry fast up until at least 12pm)

—————————————— **Afternoon** ——————————————
(get hydrating with fresh fruit or even better slow juiced fruits/berries/melons)

—————————————— **Evening** ——————————————
(aim to wind down to a dry fast by around 6pm to 7pm)

—————————————— **Night** ——————————————
(work your way up to dry fasting from the evening until 12pm the following day)

Today's Notes (Highlights, Thoughts, Feelings, What Could You Improve On?)

"Fruits have the highest healing energy frequencies among all food groups. Vegetables are the next highest. Cooked meats rank the lowest."

Today's Date:

Morning
(work towards continuing your night time dry fast up until at least 12pm)

Afternoon
(get hydrating with fresh fruit or even better slow juiced fruits/berries/melons)

Evening
(aim to wind down to a dry fast by around 6pm to 7pm)

Night
(work your way up to dry fasting from the evening until 12pm the following day)

Today's Notes (Highlights, Thoughts, Feelings, What Could You Improve On?)

"Mucus congestion (caused by dairy products) leads to a lack of mineral utilization (Calcium, Magnesium, Potassium, etc)."

Today's Date:

Morning
(work towards continuing your night time dry fast up until at least 12pm)

Afternoon
(get hydrating with fresh fruit or even better slow juiced fruits/berries/melons)

Evening
(aim to wind down to a dry fast by around 6pm to 7pm)

Night
(work your way up to dry fasting from the evening until 12pm the following day)

Today's Notes (Highlights, Thoughts, Feelings, What Could You Improve On?)

"Did you know that fruit juice (slow juiced) will offer you more Calcium than Cow's Milk?"

Today's Date:

Morning
(work towards continuing your night time dry fast up until at least 12pm)

Afternoon
(get hydrating with fresh fruit or even better slow juiced fruits/berries/melons)

Evening
(aim to wind down to a dry fast by around 6pm to 7pm)

Night
(work your way up to dry fasting from the evening until 12pm the following day)

Today's Notes (Highlights, Thoughts, Feelings, What Could You Improve On?)

"Your body will use sweating (fevers), vomiting, diarrhea, frequent urination, colds, flus, and daily elimination as means to detox a toxic state. Let it run its course."

Today's Date:

Morning
(work towards continuing your night time dry fast up until at least 12pm)

Afternoon
(get hydrating with fresh fruit or even better slow juiced fruits/berries/melons)

Evening
(aim to wind down to a dry fast by around 6pm to 7pm)

Night
(work your way up to dry fasting from the evening until 12pm the following day)

Today's Notes (Highlights, Thoughts, Feelings, What Could You Improve On?)

"Pain is merely a sign of energy blockage(s) resulting from acidosis. Alkalization is the key (through detoxification)."

Today's Date:

Morning
(work towards continuing your night time dry fast up until at least 12pm)

Afternoon
(get hydrating with fresh fruit or even better slow juiced fruits/berries/melons)

Evening
(aim to wind down to a dry fast by around 6pm to 7pm)

Night
(work your way up to dry fasting from the evening until 12pm the following day)

Today's Notes (Highlights, Thoughts, Feelings, What Could You Improve On?)

"Keep on loving! Love is alkalizing, it improves digestion and kidney elimination. Your blood and lymph flow will also improve."

Today's Date:

Morning
(work towards continuing your night time dry fast up until at least 12pm)

Afternoon
(get hydrating with fresh fruit or even better slow juiced fruits/berries/melons)

Evening
(aim to wind down to a dry fast by around 6pm to 7pm)

Night
(work your way up to dry fasting from the evening until 12pm the following day)

Today's Notes (Highlights, Thoughts, Feelings, What Could You Improve On?)

"Ensure any amalgam fillings in your teeth are replaced with composite fillings – preferably by a holistic dentist."

Today's Date:

Morning
(work towards continuing your night time dry fast up until at least 12pm)

Afternoon
(get hydrating with fresh fruit or even better slow juiced fruits/berries/melons)

Evening
(aim to wind down to a dry fast by around 6pm to 7pm)

Night
(work your way up to dry fasting from the evening until 12pm the following day)

Today's Notes (Highlights, Thoughts, Feelings, What Could You Improve On?)

"Use parsley to detox mercury out of your body."

Today's Date:

———————————— **Morning** ————————————
(work towards continuing your night time dry fast up until at least 12pm)

———————————— **Afternoon** ————————————
(get hydrating with fresh fruit or even better slow juiced fruits/berries/melons)

———————————— **Evening** ————————————
(aim to wind down to a dry fast by around 6pm to 7pm)

———————————— **Night** ————————————
(work your way up to dry fasting from the evening until 12pm the following day)

Today's Notes (Highlights, Thoughts, Feelings, What Could You Improve On?)

"Sleep is very vital for your healing. Wind down by 7pm and aim to be in bed by 10pm to 10:30pm (if possible)."

Today's Date:

Morning
(work towards continuing your night time dry fast up until at least 12pm)

Afternoon
(get hydrating with fresh fruit or even better slow juiced fruits/berries/melons)

Evening
(aim to wind down to a dry fast by around 6pm to 7pm)

Night
(work your way up to dry fasting from the evening until 12pm the following day)

Today's Notes (Highlights, Thoughts, Feelings, What Could You Improve On?)

"Keep a positive mindset. Remind yourself that everything is possible & you WILL achieve your goals"

www.ingramcontent.com/pod-product-compliance
Lightning Source LLC
Chambersburg PA
CBHW031159020426
42333CB00013B/743